Zoblit Books

Pointless
BLANK JOURNAL

A Create - It - Yourself

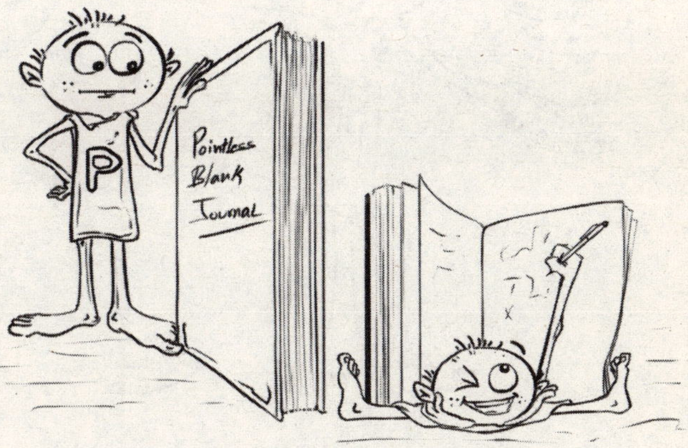

The Pointless Blank Journal

A Balanced diet publication

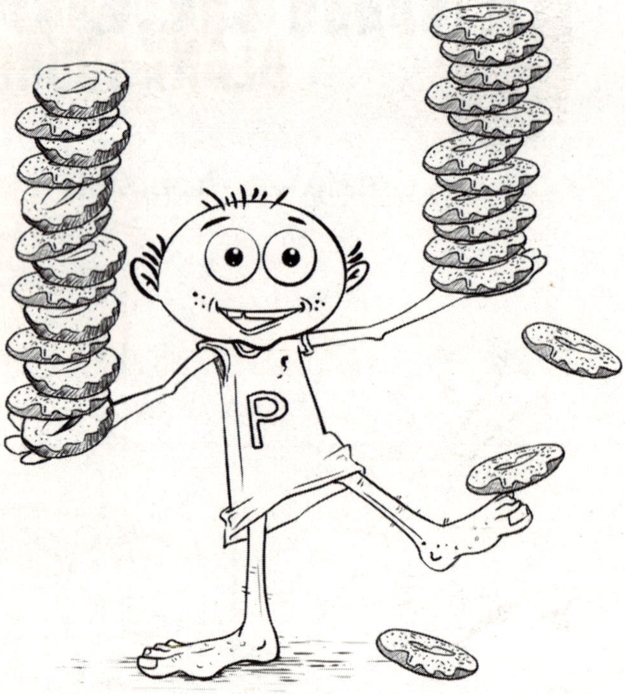

This is a monographic publication.
Apologies for those people who were expecting this Journal Book to be completely blank.
This is not the case. As the author of this book
I wish to inspire you to get writing on a single topic or issue.
We would like all participants to define a starting and an end point which can become
your overall goal to achieve. Whatever you decide to write about should be on a one-off basis.

YES THIS IS A BLANK POINTLESS JOURNAL BOOK

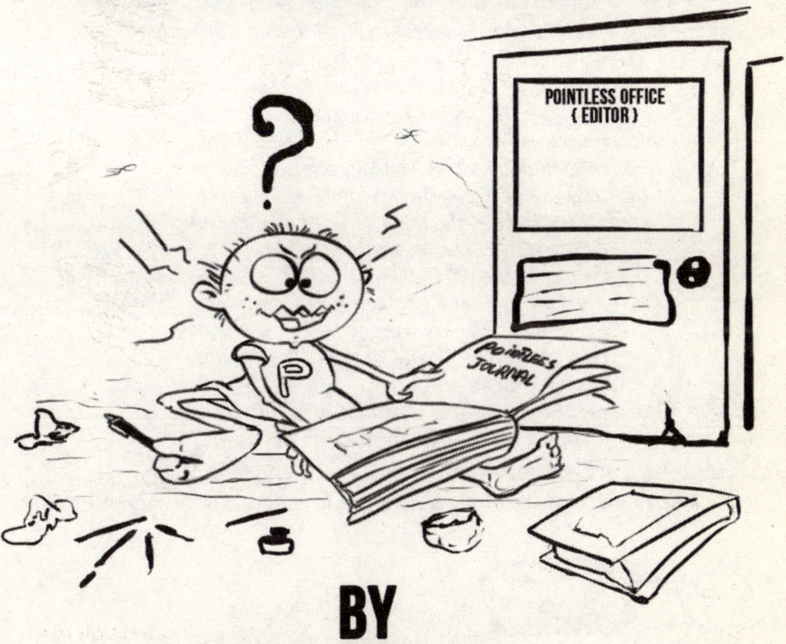

BY

YAYA NOBODY

Zoblit Books
Published by Zoblit ltd
Zoblit ltd. Unit 2 Vulcan House. Vulcan Road Leicester LE5 3EF
A Division of Nothing
Hoping to open a branch in Mars. Jupiter and the Milky Way Galaxy.

I saw a BBC Programme The Apprentice where they created
a children's book within 24hrs from start to finish.
Then friends of mine challenged me to create
15 books in 15 days and I accepted this challenge in a fun way.

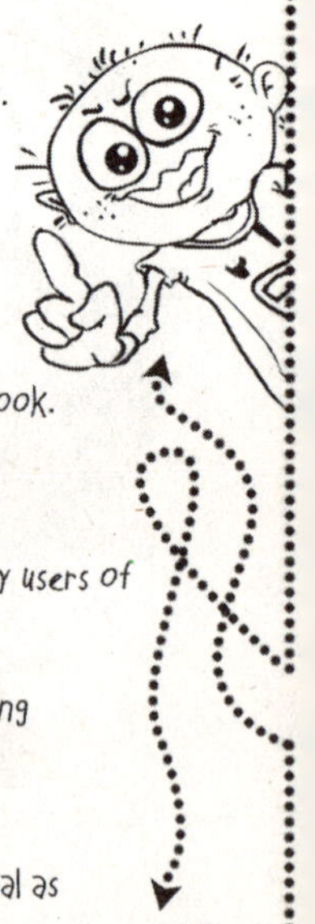

So here is my attempt to create my own books.
Seriously do people really read this small print page?
Book Created by Mr Yaya Nobody
Book Illustrated by M Nobody

To become somebody I will need to sell 1 million copies of this book.
Blank Pages Design by Yaya Nobody
Seriously you are still reading this page!!!
www.zoblit.com

Please only purchase authorised edition of this Pointless Blank Journal as
I really do want to sell 1 million copies of this book
and become Mr Somebody. So here is the deal.
You complete all the Blank pages of this Journal
and share this amongst your friend.
If they think the stuff you have written is really good
then why not send your completed journal to
Mr Nobody and if it is really good then who knows
Mr Nobody may be able to publish this for you
and you can also become Mr Somebody.

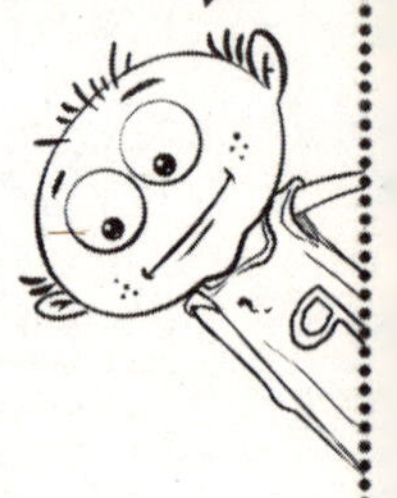

Isbn: Please insert here once your Journal is published : ....
Printed and bound somewhere in this world.
As there is not enough room to write the ISBN in font size 72 pts
on this page please check the back cover for the official ISBN of this publication

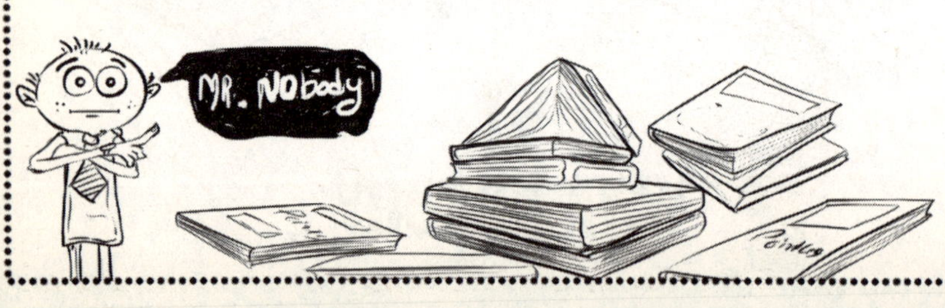

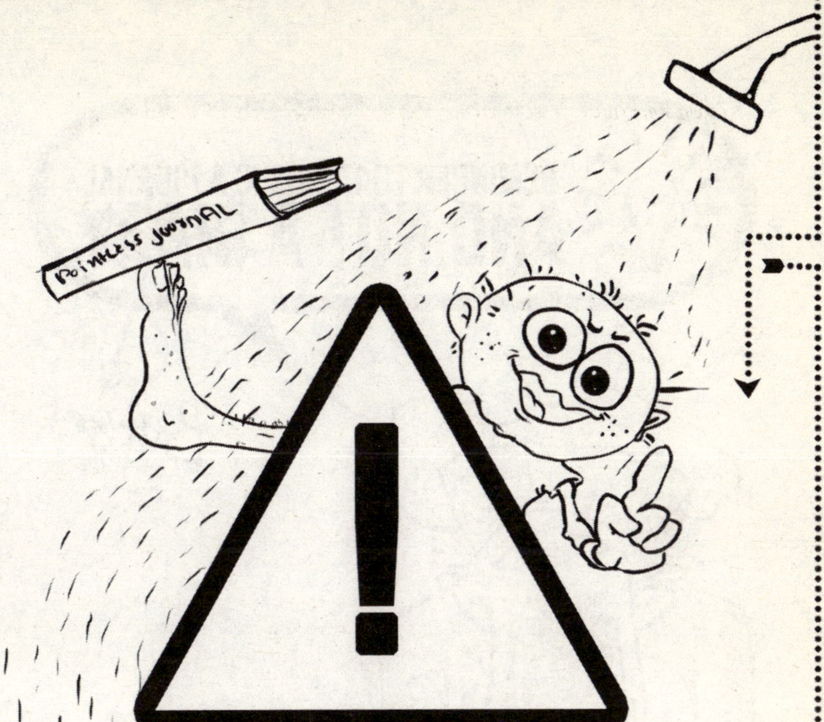

WARNING:

THIS JOURNAL IS ABOUT TO DISRUPT YOUR LIFE.
YOU MUST TAKE THIS JOURNAL WITH YOU EVERYWHERE.

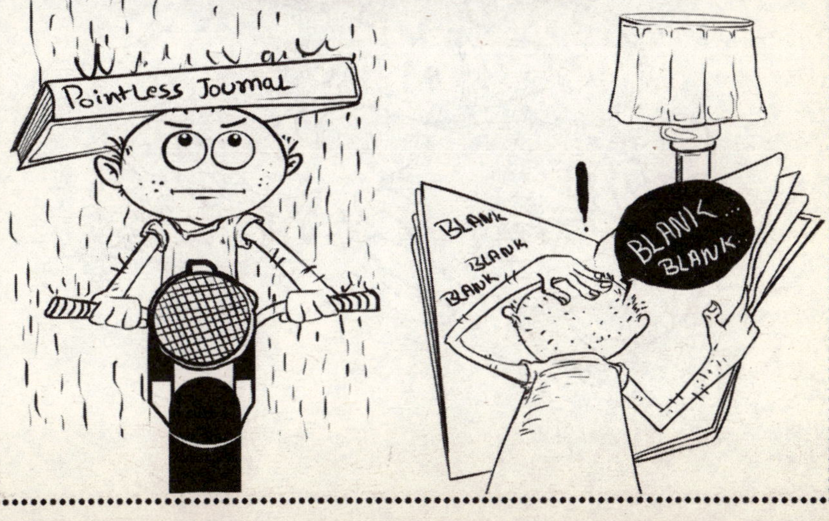

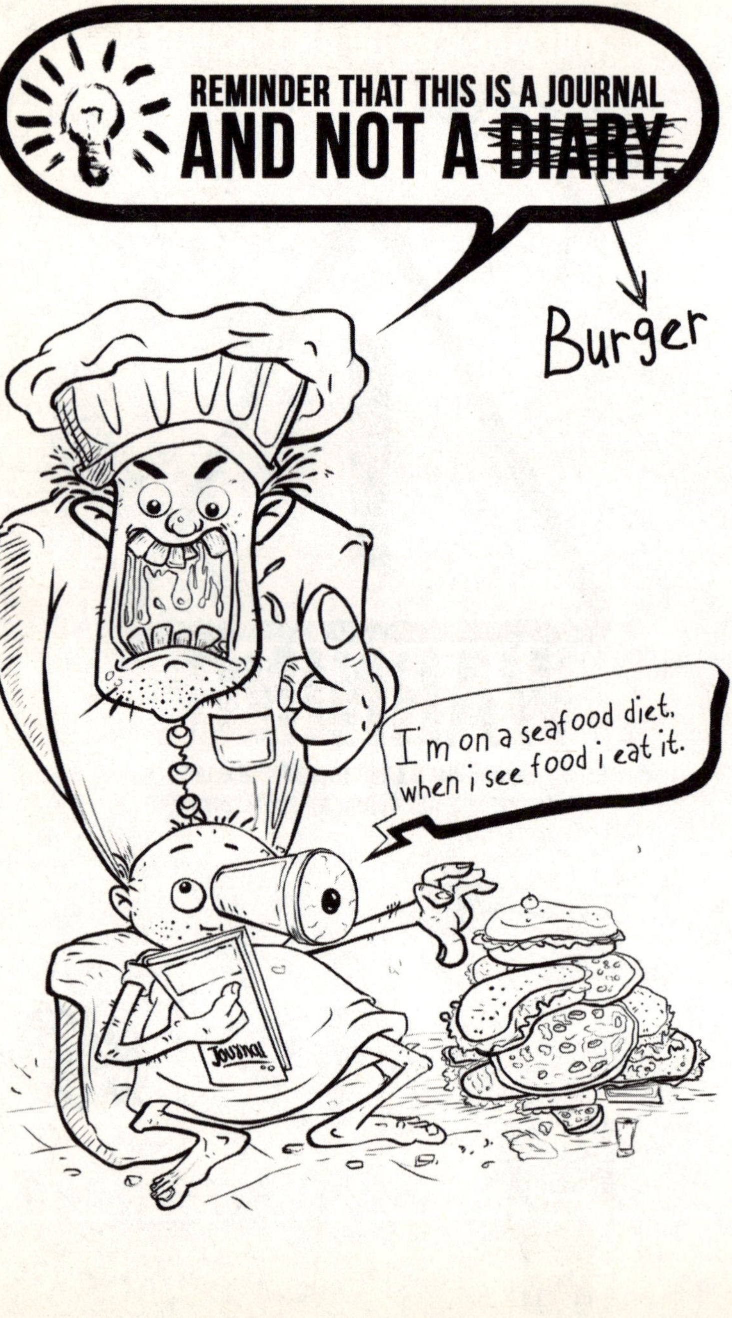
REMINDER THAT THIS IS A JOURNAL
AND NOT A ~~DIARY.~~
Burger
I'm on a seafood diet.
when i see food i eat it.
Journal

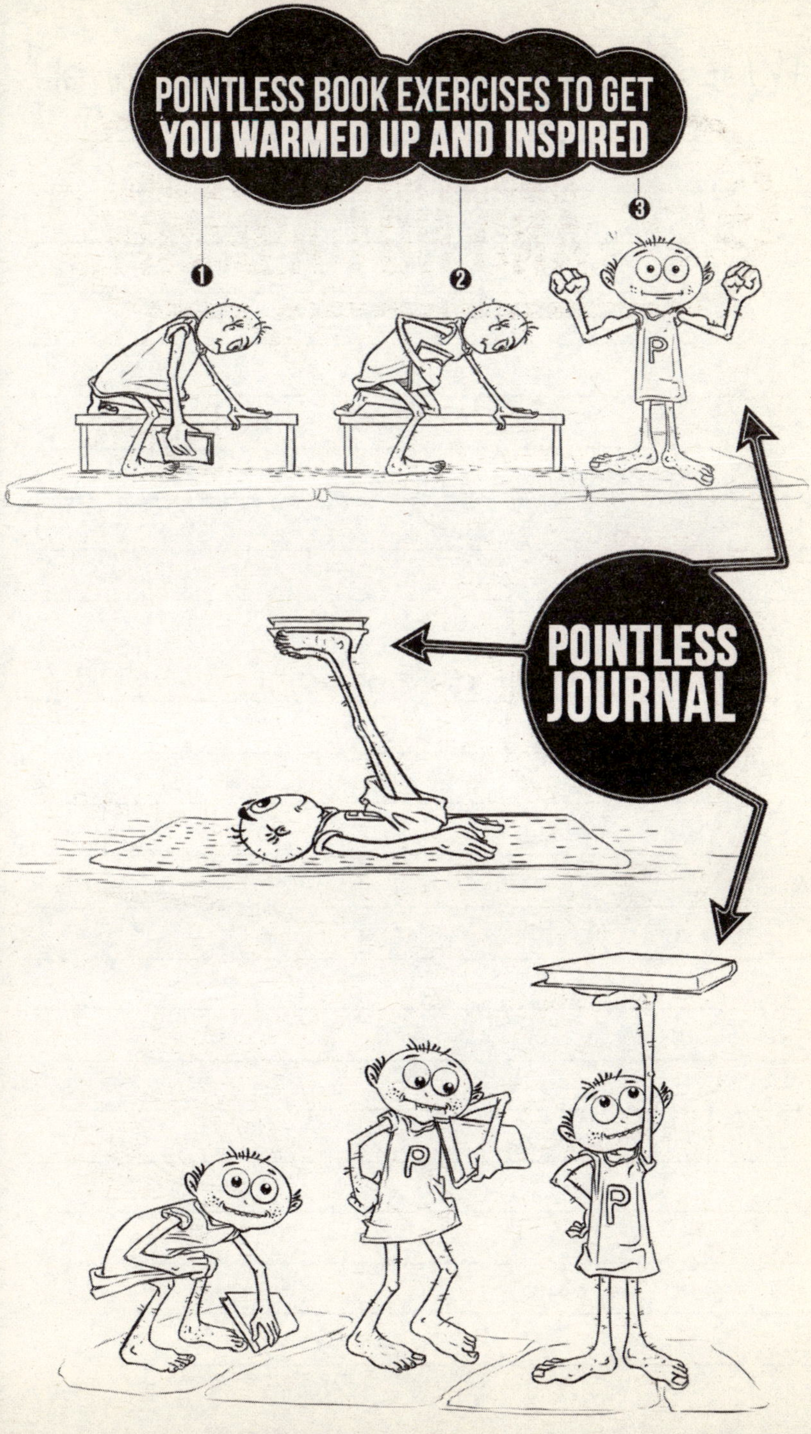
POINTLESS BOOK EXERCISES TO GET YOU WARMED UP AND INSPIRED
1
2
3
P
POINTLESS JOURNAL
P
P

What will be your purpose for using this Journal?

What will be your starting point?

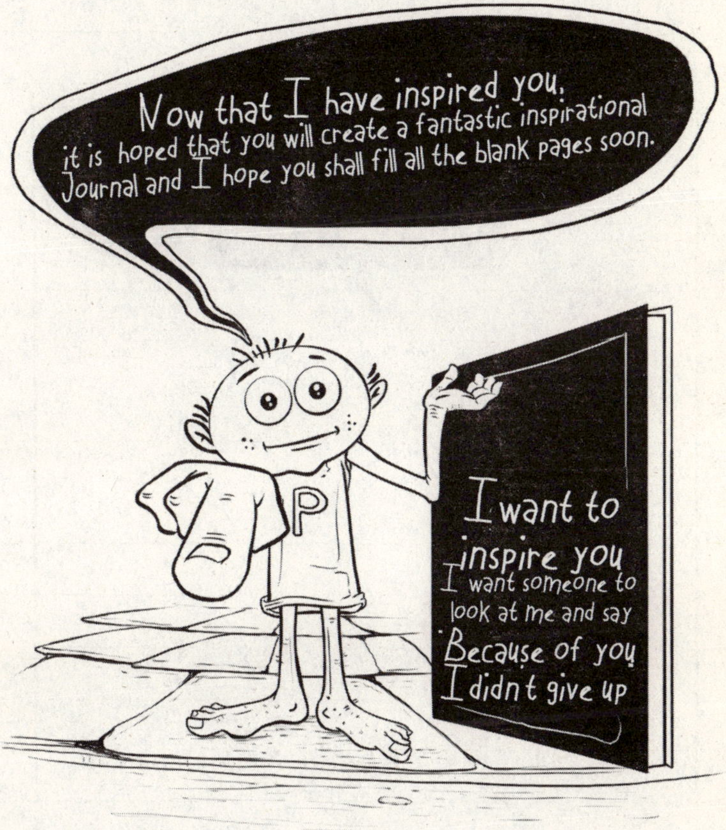
Now that I have inspired you,
it is hoped that you will create a fantastic inspirational
Journal and I hope you shall fill all the blank pages soon.
I want to
inspire you
I want someone to
look at me and say
Because of you
I didnt give up

Warning!

The rest of the pages in this Journal are Blank

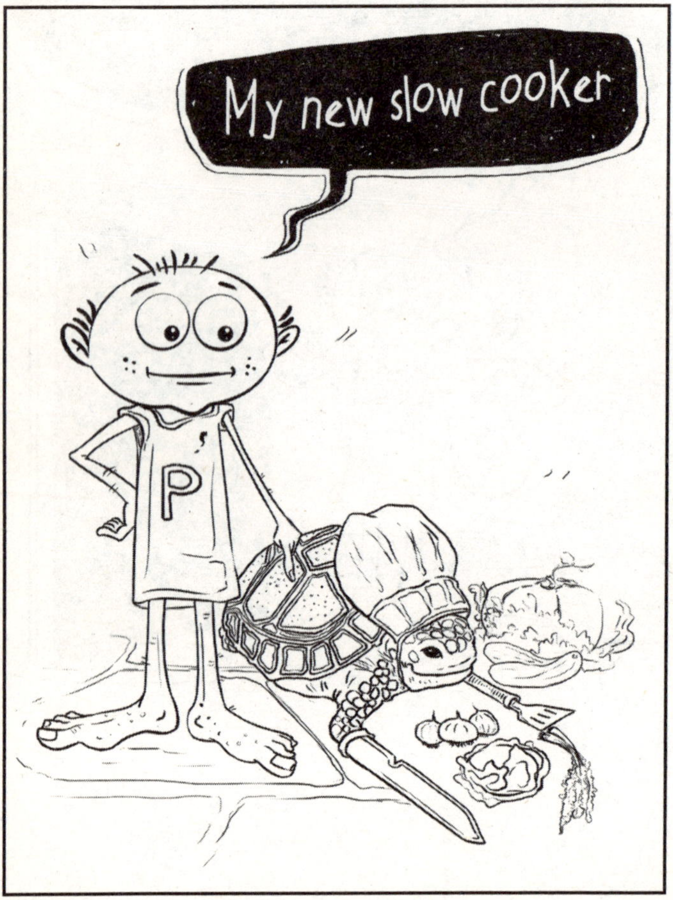